MEDITATION NOT MEDICATION

Heal Yourself Using Your Mind-Body
Connection with Healing Meditation

JENNIFER BROOKS

Meditation Not Medication: Heal Yourself Using Your Mind-Body Connection with Healing Meditation

Jennifer Brooks

Table of Contents

<u>Disclaimer</u>

Nothing in this book is intended to prescribe or to diagnose any health problem or disorder. None of the information is meant to take the place of your health care provider's advice or medical treatment.

<u>Introduction</u>

What if I told you there was a way to help heal your body, mind, and spirit that didn't involve doctors, drugs or even spiritual gurus?

On top of that, what if I said that this method of healing costs nothing and really doesn't demand much of your day? Stay with me now. I know you're ready to roll your eyes and say, "Really?" My response to that is, "Really!" Absolutely. Without a doubt.

Healing meditation asks nothing more of you than sitting for approximately 20 minutes a day in silence or visualizing your health. Nothing more. Well, if you've ever tried meditation, you may believe that's quite a chunk of time to sit "doing nothing." Then again, if you've attempted meditation and found it beneficial in any way, you know these 20 minutes are well worth the investment – even if you've only used it to renew your energy, refuel your goals or simply release stress.

Here, though, I must add a caveat. Don't use this form of meditation in place of your doctor's advice, conventional medicine or any other form of treatment—at least not at first. As you read through this book, you'll learn the simply astounding results to not only your emotional well-being, but your mental outlook as well as your physical health.

Before you embark on this health journey, discuss your intentions with your physician. He'll no doubt encourage you. The advantage to this is that when the biomarkers of your particular health problems improve, he'll have some idea why. If you don't do this, he may very well credit any medication you've been taking that up until this point that may not have even worked very well.

The History of Healing Meditation

To truly understand why healing meditation is considered so remarkable by many, you first need to understand the history not only of meditation, but more importantly of Western medicine itself.

In the Western world – Western Europe as well as North America – the typical view of treatment of disease is something that is done to the body. Physicians, for many years, saw themselves as dispensers of chemicals which stimulated the body's healing from outside itself.

Eastern medical systems such as Chinese Traditional Medicine and the Indian Ayurvedic system perceive healing as springing from within the body itself if given the proper conditions. No external, artificial stimulation is needed. It's not surprising then that many Eastern traditions, if not all of them, support various forms of meditation, including the healing varieties, while Western medicine has looked askance at it.

That is, until recently. The conventional medical community has finally taken the effort to investigate objectively the effects of healing on not only the mind and body, but also the physical body as well. As a result of this newfound open-mindedness, these intrepid investigators are also realizing another aspect of the body. At one time, many mainstream scientists believed in a split between the mind and body. The two, they believed, were two separate entities. It made little difference that the mind was contained in the body. That's why physicians treated the body as they did in times of ill health.

Recently though – within the last generation – this view is changing. More and more physicians see the evidence that the mind holds an amazing power over the body. This power is capable not only of healing, but also of influencing the body in many other ways as well. Western medicine now understands – better than it ever has before – that the mind plays a vital role in mental, emotional, and physical functions.

Believe it or not, this is a seismic shift for the conventional medical community. We're all learning – you and I included – by extension the full effects the mind exerts on our bodies. Most of us are slowly taking down that artificial veil that separated our bodies from our minds.

We're learning through experience that if you change your method of thinking, you can potentially change the direction of your life. By extension, changes in your thinking can also trigger changes in your health – physical, emotional and mental.

This is the goal of healing meditation. As with all meditation, you dwell in the moment. In this moment, you affirm that your body is whole, your thoughts are of wellness, and your emotions are void of all stress (or as some call it, "artificial stress").

Why am I so Confident in this Process?

I know that meditation can work for you if you just give it half a chance. What makes me so confident? I've seen it work miracles in my own life. Several years ago, I was faced with a serious illness. While I had been meditating occasionally, I increased the amount of time I devoted to this practice and immediately began visualizing a whole and healthy body.

My surgery was successful, my follow-up treatment equally successful, and today I'm feeling better than I ever have before. My friends are amazed at my recovery, but even more, they were astonished at the positive attitude I maintained throughout the entire journey. The doctors and nurses who treated me were also impressed with the speed of my recovery as well as my attitude.

Soon, friends were asking me how I managed it all. When I told them of my meditation routine, they wanted to know more. That got me thinking: there might be more individuals faced with physical, emotional or mental issues who could benefit from meditation, but don't know how or where to start.

If you feel that something isn't quite right in your life, then perhaps you should look at what the practice of healing meditation can do for you. You may be facing a major physical health issue as I was. Perhaps you're barraged with "stress on steroids," as many of us are these days. Or it could be any health issue in between.

Meditation has even been known to help youth with Attention Deficit Hyperactivity Disorder. If healing meditation works for all of these issues, then it certainly can help you cope with – and even heal – what's askew in your life.

The best part is that you can try it, risk free. Meditation costs you nothing. It has no harsh, unwanted side effects like some of today's powerful medications do. You can do it anywhere, anytime, if you have any issue in your life that you feel needs healed.

How Does this Book Help You

This book aims to lead you through a thorough investigation of the healing process through the practice of meditation. Below are only a few of the aspects of this subject we'll discuss:

- The definition of healing
- What it means to heal the mind, body and spirit
- Irrefutable scientific evidence of the mind healing the physical body through meditation
- The calming atmosphere meditation creates to enable the healing of the mind
- How to free yourself from the demons of anger and anxiety
- The exact elements that create a powerful healing meditation session
- The healing potential of guided imagery

In this book, you'll learn how to teach your body to heal itself as well as to prevent potential physical or emotional issues. Whether you've thought about it before or not, once you begin your healing practice you'll be truly astounded at how the mind and body work together as one to create a *whole healthy you*.

Chapter 1: Healing the Mind, Body and Spirit

Regenerating. Renewing. Reinvigorating.

These are three words that accurately describe the meditation process. You may consider this simple yet challenging act of a quiet 20 minutes as a mere reprieve from the world around you. But, as you quiet both your body and mind, you'll soon discover a more profound process is occurring during this time.

Change occurs slowly at first – at least it may seem like that to you. Then one day, after several weeks or several months of regular practice, something different happens. You react differently – dare you say more calmly – to a stressful situation; you find events that once set off an angry, even hostile response now barely get a rise out of you. Or perhaps – and this is what many consider the most dramatic – your blood pressure level has normalized, your arthritis pain has eased, or you may even notice your diabetes is easier to manage.

When you step back and view meditation from this perspective, you have to come to terms with the fact that some process isn't working within you. You might even be tempted to say meditation works on a molecular level. It's hard to say if any scientist or medical doctor would view it like this. But there is one thing most experts seem to agree on now: the meditation process can heal a wide variety of ills.

What is Healing? What is Curing?

While many have debated on the differences between the definitions of healing and curing for years, you may throw your hands up without a clue. There is, however, a fundamental difference between the two processes.

Your doctor *cures* you of an illness by providing you with a form of external treatment. In this case, the symptoms of your illness may disappear and indeed your body is restored to health. But it's just as likely that your health care provider merely treated the symptoms – the outward signals which alert your body to the fact that something is wrong. In these cases, the physical symptoms and the physical causes may indeed be removed. But that doesn't necessarily mean the deep root of the problem has been pulled out of your system.

To fully understand this, compare your physical illness to a dandelion in the middle of a beautiful yard. It's a disturbing, unsightly blotch on the body of the lawn. If you don't take care of it before the weed goes to seed, you'll have more dandelions cropping up. So, you go outside and cut the flower off the dandelion. Now, you can't see the weed and therefore it won't be able to spread. For a few days you're happy and your yard is "well."

One day, though, you walk outside and the dandelion is back. You may also discover you now have two dandelions resting together in your yard. How can that be? You pulled the weed. The flower didn't go to seed. That should have ended it all. Why didn't it? You probably already know the reason. You may have pulled the plant out, but you didn't get to the root of the problem, in this case in a very literal sense. That's basically what a cure proffered from outside of your body does. It may lessen the symptoms to make you think the illness (or dandelion) is gone, but that doesn't guarantee it really is.

Healing, however, is completely different. To continue our dandelion analogy, meditation approaches the weed differently. You guessed it. The healing process begins with the rousting of the root cause. From there, the "symptoms" associated with the problem – in this case the dandelion itself – would disappear. The good news is that you don't need to deal with a reappearance of the dandelion. The lawn is healed.

Think about this. Meditation, by its very nature, works at discovering the root of your problem whether it is of a physical nature, dealing with mental problems, or grappling with emotional issues.

But What Does Healing Really Mean?

This is all well and good, you may say, but can meditation really work at these problems that medicine and the best Western technology can't?

It seems so. More hospitals and medical doctors than ever before are expanding beyond just medications and the treatment of the symptoms of illnesses and diseases. They're inviting – and even encouraging – their patients to participate in what is now referred to as "integrative medicine." This "new" approach to medicine recognizes that physical, mental, and emotional problems are often not solved many times until other, deeper issues in an individual's life are resolved. Healing meditation is just one of these marvelous tools.

What Can Healing Meditation Do For You?

Of course, there are no guarantees that healing meditation will allow you to completely shed that blood pressure medication or eliminate your arthritis pain. But, if you allow it, it can be a contributing factor to a new, more tranquil you. That, by extension, should reduce your dependence on any number of medications.

A new, serene you is also the best method of *preventing* many disorders as well. These statements aren't just being thrown out there to seduce you into meditation; they are statements that can be backed up by statistics. A Detroit-based chemical company, for example, offered a meditation program to its employees. After three years, the results were reflected in unexpected ways.

Productivity at the company during this period skyrocketed by 520 percent. Not surprisingly, profits also increased by a remarkable 120 percent. But that's not all. This was accomplished with an 85 percent decrease in absenteeism, and the incidence of work-related injuries decreased by 70 percent.

It's been estimated that since 1930, some 1500 clinical studies have been performed noting the benefits of meditation on health. Emotionally and mentally, individuals who meditate have less anxiety overall and are less nervous. At the same time, meditators report they are more self-confident and are more independent than they had been.

Regular meditation also results in long-term physical health benefits. The ones below are just a sampling of how meditation has been known to help individuals.

- Individuals experienced lower heart rates, respiratory functions and blood pressure levels.
- Oxygen consumption decreased.
- 75 percent of insomniacs slept better.
- Individuals experienced a reduction of cortisol, the so-called stress hormone, which in turn, helped them deal with the stresses of their lives better.
- Premenstrual symptoms lessened within five short months of the initial meditation session.
- Risk of stroke and heart attack fell by an average of 8 to 15 percent.

Your body has an incredible power to balance and heal itself and meditation is one of the strongest tools you have. Allow it to renew, reinvigorate, and regenerate you. Allow it to heal your life.

Chapter 2: Thank You Dr. Benson and Dr. Ornish: Healing Cardiovascular Disease

Even though the history of meditative research extends back to the 1930s, it wasn't until the 1970s that the medical community really began taking it seriously. This about-face was due in large part to the pioneering research of then Harvard-based cardiologist Herbert Benson. His landmark book, *The Relaxation Response,* quickly caught the eye of the medical community. But moreover, the book took the public by storm.

In this book, Dr. Benson showed through undisputable controlled scientific studies that meditation, especially mantra-based meditation such as Transcendental Meditation, helped to alleviate the risks of cardiovascular disease.

This led to an exciting evolution in the treatment of disease in this country. It particularly led to changes in the way that doctors and laypeople alike viewed cardiovascular disease. Through his research, he discovered two very important aspects of meditation on the body. The first is that the quieting of the mind can really slow several aspects of your body's functions. Included in this is your heart and breathing rate. Additionally, your blood pressure can also be positively affected. For many individuals, this practice can also relax tense muscles.

The second aspect of this ancient practice is its ability to alter your brainwaves. The act of meditation actually increases the frequency of alpha waves. This classification of wave is universally recognized by the medical community as a signal of a "wakeful rest." Occurring more frequently in accomplished meditators, the presence of alpha waves indicates that the brain has momentarily abandoned its goal-oriented tasks and is entering into a state of deep relaxation – not to be mistaken with sleep.

This state, Benson confirmed, can have tremendous positive results on your health – especially your heart. His research opened an avenue that other researchers have followed. Today there's no denying the immense impact meditation can have on various disorders of the heart.

Meditation and Cardiovascular Disease

So exactly what diseases or disorders are classified as cardiovascular diseases? They actually run the spectrum of disorders that aren't considered very serious (if cared for properly) to some disorders which can quickly cause death.

Some of these include:

- Angina
- Cardiomyopathy
- Congestive heart failure
- Coronary artery disease
- Heart attack
- High blood pressure
- High cholesterol levels
- High triglyceride levels

Meditation can help all of these disorders, according to many experts. But perhaps nowhere is this more apparent than in the treatment of high blood pressure. It is believed that about 68 million people have high blood pressure today. But, of course, that's only an estimate. Many individuals have this disorder but are exhibiting no symptoms. In many cases, the first symptom is actually a heart attack. That's why high blood pressure is called the "silent killer."

A generation or two ago, this disorder was most associated with an aging population. Its demographics have changed dramatically within the last 20 years. Now, it's not unusual for youth to also experience this problem. Does this mean those youth must live the rest of their lives on medication?

Maybe not, according to one randomized clinical trial, which assessed the effectiveness of meditation on blood pressure levels. This study, published in the professional journal of Psychosomatic Medicine, examined a group of 73 healthy adolescents. The researchers divided the students into two groups. The first was a control group that did not perform meditation. The second group was asked to meditate, focusing their attention on their breath. Those students who meditated experienced significantly lower blood pressure levels as well as a slower heart rate.

Another trial examined the blood pressure levels of adults who already had developed coronary artery disease. In this study, published in the *Archives of Internal Medicine*, one of the two groups practiced a mantra-based meditation. The other group didn't meditate. The individuals who performed the meditation sessions were found to experience lower blood pressure levels than the group who didn't.

Blood pressure, though, can be a temperamental gauge. If you have problems in this area, you may already know that when you get nervous, anxious, or angry, it can spike. This causes a dilemma for your doctor – and a potentially dangerous situation for you.

If your doctor finds no way to effectively treat these spikes with the proper amount of medication, these elevated periods of blood pressure can mean a potential heart attack or stroke. But, if he writes a prescription that fails to take into account the lower blood pressure readings, your levels could drop dangerously low.

Prescribe Meditation, Not Medication

This is where the healing power of meditation comes into play. Gabriel Weiss, MD, author of *The Healing Power of Meditation,* recounts a patient he had with high blood pressure. Finally, Dr. Weiss abandoned prescribed medication in those situations where the patent would experience a spike in blood pressure. Instead, she performed a breath meditation (fully described in Chapter 7). Dr. Weiss, in essence, prescribed meditation for those incidences where the patient would definitely experience increases in blood pressure.

There was also a bonus to this experience. The patient adopted a consistent meditation program, which resulted in her actually getting upset or nervous far less often than she used to.

Meditation and an Irregular Heartbeat

One of the first thoughts that come to mind for many of us when we hear the word meditation is of the yogis who are able to slow their heart rate through this practice. You may believe that this is an exaggerated benefit. Certainly, you say, this can't be true for everyone.

Perhaps you'll never be able to lower your heart rate as low as some who have meditated for decade, but science now confirms that you can indeed lower your heart rate. If you have an irregular heart beat – especially one that beats too rapidly – you want to take special notice of the result of the following study.

This particular study was conducted by Herbert Benson. He found that those individuals who performed a mantra-based meditation like Transcendental Meditation slowed the beating of their hearts by three beats per minute.

Can Meditation Help Congestive Heart Failure?

Congestive heart failure is a weakness of the heart which contributes to an accumulation of fluid in the lungs and nearby body tissues. Could meditation help a physical condition like this? In some cases, it really can.

Sounds nearly miraculous, doesn't it? That's what many medical experts believed until the results of controlled clinical trials proved otherwise. In one six-month-long study, 23 African Americans with congestive heart failure were divided into two groups. The first group was instructed on the proper meditation techniques. They performed these faithfully for the full period of the study. The second group was given health education classes.

The group that meditated reported they experienced improvement in their overall state of well-being. Not only that, but they also experienced a verifiable increase in exercise capacity as well as fewer hospital visits than the control group.

A similar study also demonstrated amazing results. This study, published in the *American Journal of Cardiology*, involved 21 individuals suffering with coronary heart disease. Those who were taught healing meditation techniques performed better on treadmill stress tests than the control group. How much better? The results showed an improvement of nearly 15 percent.

The Ornish Plan

Up until very recently, it was a "law" in the medical community that damage inflicted by heart disease couldn't be reversed. That law seems to have recently been broken, thanks to the efforts of cardiologist Dean Ornish. His program included meditation, as well as a variety of healthy lifestyle choices. While his program is more than just meditation, this ancient practice is a large part of its success.

Is meditation a viable option for your specific symptoms of cardiovascular disease? The only individuals capable of making that decision are you and your healthcare provider. Yes, you really do need to include this professional in your decision. Remember, never reduce or stop your medication without your doctor's complete approval.

Chapter 3: Healing the Body: Cancer – A Unique Situation…Or Is It?

Many experts believe when it comes to healing cancer, the situation becomes more complicated than with heart disease. After all, for many individuals, stress is the major contributor to many forms of heart disease. Any number of variables can cause cancer, many of which the medical community doesn't even know about yet.

Some meditation experts and health care professionals caution about expecting the cancerous cells in your body to miraculously disappear after several months of meditation. This doesn't mean that it's not a valuable instrument to have and use, because it certainly is. They say that the advantages lie in meditation's ability to decrease the amount of stress you may be experiencing, and by providing you with an increased quality of life during these difficult times.

While meditation may not heal cancer directly, professionals argue that it can work on the secondary causes of cancer. In fact, it can even promote the healing of your body by working on your body's immune system. Don't give up hope, even with these words of caution. Healing your body, even in the throes of this dreaded disease, is indeed within your reach.

According to some medical specialists who advocate meditation, the benefits are threefold. First, meditation can heal you emotionally, freeing you from such demons as fear and depression, often partners in crime with cancer. Secondly, meditation helps alleviate the pain that many experience during these times as this disease plays out. Thirdly, a regular meditative program can help bolster your immune system-- your body's most powerful healing tool and often the first area compromised by not only the cancer itself, but by chemotherapy treatment as well.

Despite what some of these experts say about the complexity and realistic expectations of meditation, there's a growing body of scientific evidence that shows promise. These studies indicate that a regular, guided meditation program may aid your body in killing the destructive cancer cells. This was once thought to be impossible, but the evidence is certainly mounting and definitely hard to ignore.

The Evidence for the Healing of Cancer

An excellent example of what meditation can do is illustrated in the results of a 2002 study published in the *Journal of Psychosomatic Research.* This research showed that when individuals performed guided meditation (which we'll discuss in Chapter 8), their bodies actually created more white blood cells. Not only that, but their bodies created the cells that specialize in attacking cancer cells.

In this particular study, 25 women with early-stage breast cancer were told to meditate at least three times a week. Prior to this venture, doctors measured the amount of the white blood cells in their bodies, called lymphocytic white blood cells (you might also hear them referred to as "natural killers"). The group spent eight weeks with this meditation program before their white blood cells were again quantified. The number of "natural killer" cells actually increased by nearly 16 percent.

Meditation Stirs White Cells to Action

In a separate study conducted at the University of South Florida, guided meditation was tested on another group of breast cancer patients. This time, there were 28 women involved. The goal of the research involved not counting the amount of "natural killer" cells, but measuring their effectiveness at attacking and actually killing the cancer cells. In medical terms, this process is referred to as cytotoxicity.

The women were divided into two groups: one which meditated and the second which didn't. All participants had been diagnosed with early-stage breast cancer. None of them had yet undergone surgery. The study followed the women from prior to their surgery and four weeks following their surgery. The control group, who didn't participate in the meditation program, was given conventional medical attention. In effect, the only aspect separating the two programs was the meditation.

The final blood tests – those taken a month after surgery – showed that those who did meditate also ended up with an amazing 75 percent more activity of the "natural killer" cells. This means that their immune systems were functioning at a higher level and naturally healing the cancer. That's an impressive jump in activity, regardless of how you look at it.

Another study followed 90 individuals diagnosed with cancer – a variety of types. These individuals performed a meditative route for seven weeks. The results? More than 30 percent – almost one third of them – had fewer symptoms of stress. Approximately 65 percent experienced fewer bouts of what researchers called "mood disturbance" than those individuals who didn't meditate.

Several years ago, a meta-study of cancer and meditation was conducted. This type of study is a review of the existing literature. Its goal is to step back from the details of individual research studies in order to view the broad brushstrokes of the scientific literature at large. It's an extremely valuable tool to get a good feel of the overall direction of the existing body of evidence.

In this review, nine separate studies were compared. The consensus? Meditation delivered "consistent benefits." These include improvement in the individual's ability to handle stress, as well as a boost in a person's psychological functioning. But that's not all the good news. Individuals who meditated were also found to be better equipped to cope with the disease, generally speaking. In effect, their overall well-being improved dramatically.

This same general literature overview found a surprising added benefit. It appears that meditation may even protect an individual's cognitive powers. Often, those dealing with cancer experience a decreased ability to function in this area. The reasons for this are varied, including distress, fatigue and reduced hormone production.

Meditation, Cancer and Depression

Let's face it. No matter how you approach it, cancer can be an ordeal. Healing from cancer is a lengthy process. For many individuals the surgery comes first. Next, a series of chemotherapy or radiation treatments, or both, are performed. For some, protracted chemotherapy treatment can begin even prior to the surgery in an attempt to shrink the tumor to be able to operate on it.

It's not surprising then that many individuals dealing with this disease also tend to fall into a depression. The good news is that this secondary effect of cancer can be alleviated by a regular meditation program. The even better news is that it's no short-term quick fix. The uplifting effects of meditation stayed with individuals even three months after they completed the practice.

Can Anything Ease this Pain?

It's not unusual for those dealing with cancer to experience chronic pain. It may be due to any number of things from the presence of the cancer itself to the harshness of the treatments. It's estimated that nearly 90 percent of persons with lung cancer experience pain at some point during their illness.

Many individuals are hesitant to take – or remain – on a narcotic medication for any length of time. Not only that, but many physicians balk at prescribing narcotics for extended periods of time... Meditation can help here as well. It appears to be the saving grace on the horizon. It not only lessens the pain, but it also lessens your dependency on the drugs.

Sleep? While I'm Going Through All This?

That's exactly what many people ask themselves. Doctors try to help by prescribing sleeping aids, but for some people this just isn't a viable option. It's good to know that meditation can help you in this area as well. Multiple studies reveal persons who meditate report less cancer-related sleep problems than those who didn't.

According to the growing body of evidence, meditation appears to be growing into a powerful tool in the healing process of cancer.

Chapter 4: Healing the Body: The Mind is More Powerful than You Think

Given the previous examples, is not difficult to see the relationship between heart disease and meditation. You may even understand why meditation works well at healing cancer and allows those affected with it to live a quality life. But can meditation really work on the host of other diseases, disorders and illnesses? And if it can, by what mechanism does it work? Science, which has long been the nemesis of healing meditation, is becoming one of its greatest advocates. Many scientists are now adopting the practice specifically because of its health benefits.

Meditation seems to work on two levels. Those who have practiced it continually report on their success. "Anecdotal evidence," as these reports are called in medical circles, doesn't hold much sway in scientific circles, though. Scientists dismiss these reports for any number of reasons.

What does count – and count heavily – are the results of controlled, scientifically-run research projects, like the ones we've examined, showing the improvement in both heart disease and cancer.

It wasn't until the results of the following study were revealed that doctors began getting a glimpse into the very real mind-body connection. Personnel from both the Davis and San Francisco campuses of the University of California conducted the research.

Here's what they found: What the researchers describe as "intensive" meditation can increase an enzyme in your body known as telomerase. This enzyme is responsible for the long-term health of your body's cells. Succinctly, telomerase slows the cells' damage caused by their continual division. Every time a cell divides, it shrinks. It's this ongoing "shrinkage problem" that's responsible for the aging process. In turn, it's the aging process that's responsible for a host of what the medical community calls *degenerative diseases*.

The research involved two groups of people. The first group received intensive meditation training from a Buddhist monk. The second group didn't practice any form of quieting the mind. They continued with their normal routines. At the end of the three-month study, the telomerase levels of both groups were measured. The rates of those who meditated were approximately one-third higher than those of the control group.

But that's not the only benefit the researchers discovered. The study also revealed several psychological benefits as well, including an increased perceived control over the subjects' environments, their lives, and their surroundings, as well as a clearer vision of their purpose in life.

You may think I'm straying from the topic when I mention the *psychological* benefits, but these benefits have a physical bearing on telomerase levels (and probably up until today you didn't even know you had any!). "We have found meditation," said Clifford Saron, one of the researchers involved, "promotes positive psychological changes and meditators showing improvement on various psychological measures had the highest levels of telomerase." In other words, the higher those telomerase levels, the better you feel in general.

Meditation Speaks to Specific Problems

One of the last disorders you may expect meditation to affect is chronic fatigue syndrome. It's an ill-defined ache that you feel all over your body. The medical community has yet to determine a cause. Therefore, the medical community is at a loss of how to treat it effectively.

Until recently, that is. Using a randomized, controlled study, researchers asked those who experienced chronic fatigue syndrome to undergo mindful meditation as well as something referred to as mindfulness-based cognitive therapy. Those individuals who went through this training boosted their energy levels as well as their overall physical activities.

Meditation and Contagious Disease

Remember the last time some virus ran through the office, or maybe through your family? It got passed from one person to the next. You might have even felt that you got it twice. Bet you weren't practicing meditation at the time. How do I know? Listen to the powerful results of this study.

The two most common types of these easily transmittable health issues are upper respiratory infections and viral intestinal infections. You no doubt are well aware of the symptoms of each.
In addition to the physiological problems, you may also experience some emotional despair as well. It could be as simple as, "Why me?" or even, "I feel so badly I could just die." We've all been there.

Meditation may not be able to replace your need for medication in these situations, but it can help lift that veil of despair. In fact, regular meditation can even replace that "low down" feeling with one of calmness and serenity. It can also help you look with an increased confidence toward your eventual recovery.

Can't Sleep? Toss the Sleeping Aids Out!

Who among us hasn't experienced at least one night of lost sleep? Some statistics cite that as many as 30 to 50 percent of the population has occasional sleep problems. There are also more individuals than you think who have chronic sleeping problems. Perhaps you're one of them. Many times we turn to either prescription or over-the-counter medications.

You may think that these aids would solve the problem. After all, there are more than enough kinds on the market – both prescription and over-the-counter. Not only that, but many people don't even hesitate to take them. Still, people lose sleep and, worse yet, the very drugs they take to help lull them into a peaceful slumber may come with a host of side effects that run the gamut from annoying to dangerous.

Meditation can help in this area too. A controlled study was conducted which involved both breast and prostate cancer patients. It showed, beyond a shadow of a doubt, that those who practiced mindful meditation, preferably lying in bed prior to retiring for the evening, slept better.

Another study involved sleep-onset insomnia, in which patients have trouble actually falling asleep, but sleep fine after that. Individuals who meditated experienced an overall 77 percent decrease in the time it took them to fall asleep compared to the control group who didn't meditate.

Can Meditation Really Help Improve Asthma?

If you suffer from asthma, then you know exactly what a severe attack feels like. It is, without a doubt, one of the scariest experiences a person can ever encounter. Your wind is abruptly curtailed. Without the ability to breathe properly, you feel as if you're about to die – literally. It's a definite feeling of suffocation.

You may have already drawn a connection between this respiratory disorder and stress. An asthma attack is exacerbated by fear or anxiety. It may not surprise you, then, to learn that many individuals with asthma have already benefitted from meditation.

One study specifically examined a group of individuals who had mild to severe asthma attacks that couldn't be controlled through treatment with conventional medication. These persons were divided into two groups for the purposes of the research. The first group received drug treatment alone. The second group received the conventional treatment, plus they were taught to meditate.

Those individuals who meditated discovered the drugs were actually more effective at controlling their asthma attacks. If you're asthmatic, you may never be able to toss your drugs out the window, but it's reassuring to learn there is a method by which they can be much more effective.

These are only a few of the many disorders that have been verified through strict scientific measures to be helped by meditation. Some of the others include:

- Chronic Obstructive Pulmonary Disease (COPD)
- Hyperventilation Syndrome
- Menopausal Issues
- Osteoarthritis
- HIV/AIDS
- Irritable Bowel Syndrome (IBS)
- Heartburn

If you're suffering from physical health issues, you may want to seriously consider trying your hand at meditation. If it doesn't actually heal your health problem, you'll at least be able to view it from a completely new perspective. Sometimes that's all it takes.

Chapter 5: Healing the Mind: Calming Words and Calming the Mind to Ease Anxiety and More

Did you see that? It seemed as if it went past at 75 miles per hour. Look there! Another one moving at the speed of light!

"Are these vehicles?" you ask. Hardly. These are the events of our lives. Thanks to technology, they move faster than ever before. The only problem is that there are times when we're left standing in the dust, wondering what just sped by.

That's not all we contend with in the twenty-first century. There are the myriad of distractions, affecting all of our senses. The ever-present television set that seems to be turned on all the time, blaring at us 24 hours a day. Noises from the internet, MP3 players, cell phones, smart phones, buzzing advertisements—they all have their effect on our minds and bodies.

Meditating Sadness Away

Sadness. You can't call it depression, but it doesn't look anything like happiness either. Sometimes we call it "the blues." You may be experiencing it as a natural response to an event in your life. You didn't receive that promotion you thought you were a shoe-in for. You didn't get the job you interviewed for. Or perhaps you're just in the "winter doldrums." You know it's not a serious depression, but you want nothing more than for it to pass. It's almost as if a sad feeling has taken hold of you and you have no control over it.

Here's where meditation can, indeed, be healing. You'll no doubt find that your "blues sessions" are shorter and less intense when you meditate regularly. That's good on paper you say, after you've meditated for several weeks. But let's face it, when that event blindsides you, it still brings you down. What do you do when you get slammed with misfortune?

Your immediate response, of course, is sadness. But you naturally don't want to allow that sadness to linger for very long, thinking it has found a permanent residence within you. This is when a short "mini-meditation" is in order. When you find yourself slipping into that state of sadness, whether it's a reaction to a known and tangible cause, like a flat tire, or to no discernible cause at all, stop.

That's right. Stop what you're doing. Stop thinking for a few moments. You're probably thinking negative thoughts, trying to figure out where to point the blame: "Why do these things always happen to me?" "It's downhill from here."

If you're like most of us, you have a million of those negative-invoking sayings inside of you just ready to burst through. Instead of running through all of them, take control of your thoughts. Don't allow the negative ones to run rampant and stampede your mind.

Stop long enough to calm your mind. Take three full meditation breaths. That's it. That's really all it takes to stop your mind from careening out of control and taking the plunge into an even deeper sadness. If your blues are from an inexplicable source or you've had a series of unfortunate events befall you, think about increasing the amount of time you spend in your meditation sessions. Some experts suggest that when you're up against tough times, you should double the length of your sessions.

If you normally spend 10 minutes a day meditating, then add another 10 to make it 20. You can do this in two ways. You can either do one 20-minute session or you can meditate two times a day, each for 10 minutes. You'll be surprised how quickly "the blues" passes you by. If you can't commit to 20 minutes, expand your session by as many minutes as you feel comfortable with. Any amount of time, actually, will help.

Anxiety: Waiting for the Other Shoe to Drop

Perhaps we're so used to "bad things" happening to us, that we just expect them. Many individuals do. When they have a series of good events, they have to say something like, "Well, this can't last forever, something bad is going to happen soon." Or some people say, "My luck is sure to run out soon."

That sinking feeling you carry with you, thinking something bad is waiting around the next bend, is called *anxiety*. Do you feel anxious for no apparent reason? I lived with a generalized inexplicable anxiety for years when I was younger. I was so accustomed to "bad things" happening to me that my mind just anticipated the next disaster. Then, I discovered meditation. It didn't take long for that anxious feeling to flee and to be replaced by a calm, optimistic outlook.

You don't have to take my word for it. Jon Kabat-Zinn recorded the results of one of his studies that showed just that. Meditation can sweep anxiety out of your mind. In Kabat-Zinn's study, twenty-two individuals with generalized anxiety and panic attacks were taught to meditate. They did so for three months. At the end of this period, 20 of them reported significantly less anxiety.

In a related study, researchers divided individuals who experienced anxiety into three groups. The first group was used as the control group. These individuals were told not to alter their usual routine. The second group received meditation training and was told to meditate daily. The third group participated in standard, conventional relaxation exercises.

The members of the groups who meditated and performed relaxation exercises were less anxious by the end of the study. The researchers said, though, that meditation may have the edge in the clearing of anxiety because it "may be more specific in its ability to reduce distractive and ruminating thoughts and behaviors."

Depression: Meditation Can Help, But . . . .

Anxiety and the blues are certainly health issues you say. But what if you have full-blown, major depression? It's been medically diagnosed as that and you're taking prescription medication for it. There's no way, you believe, that something as simple as meditating can help you.

Don't think for a second that I would ever advise you to trade your medication in for a meditation bench and a candle. That's not going to happen. That doesn't mean, though, that you can't alleviate the symptoms of your depression through a solid meditation program. Many individuals who suffer with major depression find it's difficult, if not impossible, to concentrate or focus on any one thing for any appreciable length of time. You can see where this would be a challenge in attempting a meditation program.

This is exactly why you're not going to stop taking those antidepressants. These drugs, in effect, replace the neurotransmitters you need to keep depression at bay. You can, however, augment that treatment. Wait until your medications have fully taken effect and your mood is lifting. Once the drugs are doing their job, you'll discover your concentration has returned. Then you can consider beginning a meditation routine.

Meditation, for many individuals, may be the treatment of choice for certain health problems. Seldom though is it the only therapy you should be using. Major depression is just one example of this. We've already talked about the role of meditation in cardiovascular disease as well as cancer.

No one would ever advise you to stop your chemotherapy to just sit and "meditate the cancer away." No one would advise you from undergoing surgery in the first place to remove the tumor. Meditation, though, can greatly enhance the healing of both of these physical disorders, and so it is with depression. I can't repeat this enough: *Don't stop taking your medication once you begin meditating.* Both avenues of treatment are needed and they pack a heck of a wallop at knocking out depression.

Give Your Feelings the Time They Deserve

Modern society discounts sadness as well as other feelings, such as anxiety and depression. It tries to downplay or even ignore them. "Snap out of it," well-meaning people tell us. When someone tells us to *give these feelings the time they deserve*, it seems inappropriate. According to many, these feelings don't deserve our time or attention at all.

Stephen Bodian, a noted meditation expert, explains that if you sit down to meditate, you need to be aware of these feelings without being judgmental. This means that you should mindfully meditate on them. As you sit, think about your "blue feelings" or your anxiety, but instead of telling yourself it's a silly or superfluous feeling, hold it lovingly in your thoughts.

The best way to begin is by becoming aware of your senses. In what parts of your body do you feel this emotion? Does your heart feel heavy? Are there any other areas which feel constricted or even choked off because of this sadness? Some individuals, after meditating on their sadness, report they feel as if they're about to cry, but can't. There are times when crying over a situation is cathartic. If meditating can bring you to the point where you can cry, don't be afraid to.

Next, become aware of your thoughts. Don't judge them. Don't dismiss them as unfounded. Just examine them. Especially take note of any sensation which may be fueling the sadness, anxiety or depression. Now is also a great time to pull up memories and images associated with these feelings. Of course, once again, you'll do this in a nonjudgmental way. It may be that you're continually replaying the same negative thoughts. This is the time to examine them without berating yourself for them. Then release them. Allow them to go free. You may discover during this process that you're crying. Allow yourself to do this as well. Too often our society tells us "not to cry over spilled milk." This can be a very beneficial action.

When I was first told do meditate on my sadness, I was a bit fearful. I felt I would only be fueling the fire. I thought I would emerge from my meditation even more depressed than when I entered it. I was surprised to find that wasn't the case. In fact, the opposite occurred. I learned that the sadness wasn't as powerful as I built it up to be. I also discovered it isn't an endless feeling. I had believed that I would never overcome it. Eventually, with the help of meditation, I did.

I must confess, though, that I have a series of dialogues I run through my head. They're the same stories I play over and over again. They're the same stories I've been playing for decades. I always seem to choose one particular "story," reminding myself of the injustice done to me. I'm sure you have a personal experience similar to this.

You may try to resolve this, only to discover that these thoughts insist on returning. Renowned meditation teacher Jack Kornfield calls these "insistent visitors." You continue to think about them because for some reason, the event remains unfinished – even if you don't recognize it. Providing these stories with the platform and expression they need can help release them. It may be the incident is more complex than it appears. The idea is not to scoff at the thoughts or even turn them away, but to gently and carefully examine them and come to terms with them.

Sometimes, you just can't rid yourself of them. You're not failing at meditation if you've noticed that even after your efforts, the habits keep re-appearing. Here are a few ways you can effectively deal with these recurring thought patterns:

1. Deal directly with your feelings

I can hear you now: "If I could do that, I wouldn't be sitting here meditating!" You're absolutely right. This, though, is anything but a quick fix. You may very well need to come to terms with your feelings before the pattern will actually leave you alone. This may mean you thoroughly need to investigate your feelings. It could be that right now you're viewing the sadness, anxiety or even depression as an iceberg. You see the 10 percent of the problem that's above the water, but you're ignoring the 90 percent below the surface.

You may believe you're spending quality time exploring all of your feelings. At some point, though, you need to ask yourself, "What feelings haven't I felt?" Don't be afraid to ask this question, like I was afraid to do for the longest time. Delving deeply into your feelings won't invite them to stay with you forever (like I thought!) or make them appear to loom larger than what you think they should be. In reality, looking below the surface enables these feelings to move along, so you can pay more attention to the rest of your life.

2. Name that feeling

Not only name it, but number it. Until you can get to the point that you can escort those sad and anxious feelings out once and for all, try this technique. You're well aware of what your most "popular" story lines are. Name them. Number them. When they float through your mind in the midst of a meditation, immediately identify them by number and allow them to float along their way. "Oh, that's story line number 3. I know it well." Then send it on its way.

3. What you resist persists

Have you ever noticed that the more you resist something – anything – you seem to draw it closer to you? It not only magnifies, but it seems as if it attracts related thoughts as well. Is this what's happening with your sad or depressing story lines? Could it be you've intentionally been holding on to these stories for a reason?

Do you think it's to your advantage to keep parading these stories out in front of your mind? Think about it before you answer. Be open to the fact that it just might be to your advantage. If so, what could be the benefits you're receiving? This is a question only you can answer.

4. Digging for the story

"There's gold in them there hills!" That was a popular saying during the Gold Rush of 1849 in California. Sure, there was gold – and lots of it – but you had to dig for it. The gold didn't just appear at your feet. What does this have to do with your negative emotions? More than you may think.

"There's gold in them there feelings!" Just like during the gold rush, there's a treasure within your sad feelings. And just like the gold, it won't appear at your feet. You'll have to dig for it. There very well could be wisdom in your sadness, depression, or anxiety. The reason these feelings won't leave could be because they're trying to teach you a deeper lesson. They won't leave until you discover it.

Do you experience the same uncomfortable, even nagging feeling during your meditation? Why not try allowing it to truly express itself? Try this exercise. You may feel uncomfortable doing this at first, but you'll soon discover it's a quite effective technique. Talk to these feelings as if they were a close and trusted friend.

Ask your feelings, "Are you trying to send me a message or teach me a lesson?" "What am I supposed to be listening for?" Then meditate on that. Sit quietly waiting for an answer. Don't rush the process. You just may find that the "dirt," in the form of sad or anxious feelings, may be covering a fortune of gold nuggets – invaluable lessons that can transform your life if you allow them.

Meditating on your depression, anxiety, or sadness is by no way a quick fix. It won't instantly "cure" the blues and have you dancing away your day. But it can yield some valuable insight to the cause of your feelings. This, in turn, can mean you'll be able to see the light at the end of the tunnel.

Chapter 6: Calming the Wild Beast: Handling Anger through Meditation

Feeling Angry?

Stop. Count to 10.

Waiting for more advice? At some point in your life, your mother, your grandmother or some other sweet and kind maternal figure may have given you these instructions. By counting to 10, the anger magically left you. On the other hand, you may have had a father, grandfather or other robust male role model tell you the best way to deal with your anger was to just let whoever was making you mad "have it." In other words, just get your anger out in the open.

Whose advice did you take? I usually ended up counting to 10, not feeling any less angry, but walking away before I let the individual "have it." Counting to 10 really didn't help me. It may never have helped you. What do you do after you count to 10 and still feel angry? Nobody ever answered that question for me. If that really worked, people still wouldn't be searching for an effective method to handle their anger.

This example vividly illustrates the role of anger in our society. It is, without a doubt, a double-edged sword. On the one hand, not expressing anger is highly valued. It's a badge you can wear that certifies you have your emotions under control. On the other hand, expressing your anger, most experts agree, is healthy. Repressed anger can not only cause you emotional pain and angst, but it can also harm you physically. So what's a person to do with his anger these days? Keep it in a jar with the lid tightly twisted on or let it roam free?

You can also count on one other fact with anger. When friends and family discover you meditate, they'll be appalled if you ever show signs of anger in front of them. They may expect certain stereotypical behavior from you, including a belief that you never get angry. So, if they do view your anger, they're stunned. Their first response may be a wisecrack like, "I see you didn't meditate today?"

The Two Sides of Dealing with Anger

The paradox of anger is that on one hand, in a "civilized society," we aren't supposed to show our anger. Yet, for the sake of our psychological – and physiological – well-being, we must also vent it in some manner. Talk about walking a tight-rope.

In reality, the relationship between anger and meditation is quite tense at times and definitely complicated. In the end, it comes down to the question of whether you're meditating on it or just repressing it.

The Relation Between Anger and Self-Talk

Many psychologists and other health-care professionals now view anger as being intimately related to negative self-talk. We all do this occasionally, especially when events or situations don't seem to be working in our favor. We may even start out by saying, "They are all against me" – whoever "they" may be.

You may even believe – as many of us have from time to time – that the entire world is against you. We usually don't hold this view for very long—but while we do, it very often appears as anger boiling up within us. Repeatedly talking to yourself in negative or even antagonistic terms can take any anger you may be feeling to a more intense level.

You can easily see how this happens, simply by thinking back to the last time you were angry. Did someone exacerbate the situation by showering you with even more negative and antagonistic words? Your anger probably escalated rapidly. On the other hand, consider the result of someone who views your anger and attempts to calm you with positive speech. Many times, the result is that your anger subsides.

Same Principle, Different Voice

When you talk to yourself when you're already angry, it's the same principle at work. The only difference is the voice you're hearing. It's your own. Meditation offers a number of ways for you to begin a gentle, loving conversation with yourself to dissolve or dispel at least some of your anger.

To that end, a meditation technique has been developed that may help you resolve the issue. Its goal is help you effectively become aware of your anger and the sensations that accompany it. Many individuals who are carrying unresolved anger never stop to ask themselves questions like: "How does it affect me physically?" Anger, just like depression and anxiety, produces physical symptoms and feelings. Too often we're in the middle of these emotions and fail to be aware of the physical traits that accompany them.

You may need to summon up a bit of courage to perform this meditation. When you first begin, it may seem as if you're stirring up your anger and allowing it to go rampant. For this reason, you need to promise yourself you won't act on this anger during the meditation and for a good length of time afterward.

This may very well be the first time you've ever truly examined your anger. The following meditation is a mindful one, just as when we talked about meditating on sadness. Allow your anger to surface, but you're going to only be aware of it. You'll view it non-judgmentally. Your ultimate goal is to be able to view this anger as if it were occurring to someone else. You simply observe it from a detached perspective.

Start by sitting or lying comfortably. Center yourself. Take several deep breaths. Relax all parts of your body. Then, you're going to become aware of the areas of your body most affected physically by the anger. Many individuals describe anger physically as being hot. Are there areas of your body that feel hot?

Others say anger has a numbing effect on their body. By that I mean there's an absence of physical feeling in the areas most affected by the anger. Mentally scan your body for this. Throughout your examination, try not to focus on the initial cause of your feelings. Set that aside. Instead, just continue to discover what the anger *feels like*.

Meet Your Anger in Your Breath

The next part of this meditation may sound strange. It may also take you some time to be able to completely accomplish it. Don't get worried if it takes you a while to adjust to this.

Inhale with the purpose of "meeting" your anger in your breath. Yes, I know it sounds like nothing you've ever done before. It's not an act that's readily describable with words. Once you've accomplished it, though, you'll know exactly what it means.

Continue with this practice. At first it will appear as if nothing is happening. But at some point you'll know when your anger meets your breath. There'll be practically no separation between the two. This is exactly why you must promise yourself not to act on the anger during this session. Eventually, the awareness you've cultivated will have your anger and your breath both existing side by side.

Breathe your anger until you feel you can handle it with some ease. In essence, the goal of this mindful meditation is to become friends with your feelings of anger. In this way your anger becomes a part of you. You're breathing your anger non-judgmentally.

You may have to practice this throughout several sessions. The ultimate goal is to gain insight into your feelings. Your aim is to be able not only to identify and live with anger, but to understand why you're feeling it. This is the first step in eliminating the need for it. Once you thoroughly understand why you feel the way you do, you then can take the necessary steps to adjust your thinking.

It may very well be that the anger you're feeling for a specific individual or a particular situation is based less on the person or the event. It could be that a trigger or set of triggers (inciting events) are related to that behavior or venue that caused the anger.

If you decide to perform this meditation, keep in mind that you'll be actually calling forth anger you may have kept locked up for a long time. You must perform this meditation with care and be sure you're ready to deal with whatever you find lying within you. The eventual benefits, however, of this particular meditation are well worth the time you invested.

Chapter 7: Elements of a Healing Meditation

"How difficult could meditation be?" you might be thinking. There's nothing to it.

In many ways you're right. You could sit down right now and meditate. Without a doubt, you'll gain many benefits. But knowing the three important elements of a productive meditative session can help you gain even more from the practice. When it comes to a meditation to help you heal, you'll want to do everything within your power to ensure you're getting the most benefit from each breath.

That's exactly what this chapter focuses on: the three most important elements of meditation. Yes, these three elements are important for any successful meditation, but play an even bigger role when you're using meditation to heal.

What are the three elements? Breath, posture, and mantra. As you progress in your meditative journey, you'll discover that the more you know about these aspects of the process, the more powerful your benefits will be.

Meditation: The Breath of Life

There's no way you can underestimate the vital connection between an effective meditation session and a healthy deep breathing routine. In every language, across all cultures and for thousands of years, breath has been synonymous with life, as it should be. If you can't breathe, your body is denied its ultimate form of nourishment.

Along the same lines, if you normally breathe shallowly, your body is receiving nourishment, but perhaps not as much as it should be. Meditation specialists say that your mind will not only become clearer, but also more tranquil as you deepen your breathing pattern.

As you focus on your breath, you'll be cementing the connection between your body and your mind. Here are some quick and easy steps to get you started on your road to healing meditation.

So You Think You Know How to Breathe?

Are you sure you're breathing at your full capacity? You may be surprised to learn you're not. Few of us actually breathe effectively without some teaching and practice. Since breath is such a vital aspect of any form of meditation, it's wise to know how to take a full and refreshingly healthy breath. The following test can tell you if you are – and help you develop this essential activity.

To take a breath that truly fills your lungs, you need to learn to breathe from your diaphragm. This isn't very complicated. It just takes some time to help your body adjust to the new habit.

It's best if you're alone for this exercise because it involves baring your abdomen. You'll also need a book. Lie on your back on the floor. Place the book on your bare stomach. If you're breathing properly, that is from your diaphragm, the book will move in rhythm with your breathing.

The diaphragm is best described as a layer of muscle which extends across the bottom of your ribcage. It actually separates your lung and heart from your abdominal cavity. Your goal is to inhale and have your diaphragm doing the work of filling your lungs with air. There is a distinct physiological advantage to this. When your diaphragm works, then your lungs are really filled to capacity. Right now, you may take a deep breath only to say that your lungs are filled with air. But if that breath didn't originate below your rib cage, there's still room for more air.

Take a deep breath through your nose. Visualize the air being pulled to the area just below your breast bone. This may take you a few tries to do, but you'll eventually accomplish it. When you're breathing from your diaphragm, you'll notice three things. First, regardless of how deep of a breath you're taking, your shoulders won't move. Second, your chest actually moves ever so slightly. Finally, the book sitting on your stomach (No, I didn't forget it was there!) moves in rhythm with your breath.

As you inhale, your stomach will rise. As you exhale, your stomach and the book will fall. Perform this activity as many times as you feel you need to. Don't hesitate to do it several times throughout the day if you like.

When you enter a meditative session, you may want to consider lying down at first with a book on your stomach to gauge your breathing. If you prefer a sitting meditation, you can place your hand on your stomach to ensure it is rising and falling properly. If you find you've lapsed into your former breathing pattern, simply place your full attention on your diaphragm and your breath. Don't be surprised if you have to concentrate on breathing through your diaphragm. This is not what your body is accustomed to doing, and it may take a bit to adjust yourself to it

Now, Let's Talk More About Making Your Breath Work for You

First, sit upright, preferably in a chair. Inhale deeply, then release it through an exhale. As you do this, notice as much as you can about what is occurring during this short period of time. Especially take notice of the air as it enters your nostrils and fills your lungs.

Some individuals pay the closest attention to the falling and rising of the breath on their abdomen. As you perform this exercise more, you'll naturally be attracted to some aspect of your breathing routine. Regardless of what you choose, it'll be the perfect area for your purposes.

Once you get accustomed to this exercise, you may want to practice breathing in a slightly different way. You may find that this is particularly beneficial at times. In this variation of breathing, you'll be introduced to the effects and inherent benefits of heavy breathing. This is different from the deep breathing we recently discussed.

The heavy breathing exercise is more like the type of breathing performed by those who hyperventilate. The beauty of this particular form is that it can momentarily stop you from thinking—by stimulating, if only briefly, a deep and relaxing meditative-like state.

To test this type of breathing pattern, seat yourself upright in a chair. Now take approximately ten rapid, but deep breaths. To follow this, you'll purse your lips and slowly, very slowly, exhale. When many individuals perform this exercise, especially for the first time, they find that they get lightheaded for a short time. That's the initial impression at least. Shortly after this, you'll probably then become keenly aware of the pleasurable act of not thinking.

That's right. Your mind may try to convince you otherwise, but *not thinking* for a few moments can actually be quite enjoyable. This experience will be linked with a very sharp awareness of yourself or your surroundings.

You may even call this a peaceful feeling. For those of you who have never meditated, this may be quite an unusual feeling. You'll also be disappointed, for within a short time, that indescribable tranquil feeling will leave you. Don't worry about this though. The whole point of this exercise is to introduce you to the peaceful, calming effects meditation can create in your life through merely focusing on your breath.

Yes, breathing is a vital element of any meditation session, but even more so when it comes to healing meditation.

Your Parents Were Right... Again: The Importance of Posture

Sit up straight, your father always told you. Well, at least my father always told me that, and he never meditated a day in his life. But his words were wise. There's no way you can harness this marvelous power of breath if your body isn't aligned properly to allow the flow of air to course through it. That's why specific meditation postures are recommended. When you're sitting in a certain fashion, it's much easier – almost second nature, in fact – to maintain a straight spine.

The most widely known position, if not notoriously the most difficult, is called the full lotus. In this position, it's recommended that you sit on the floor, not on a chair or a couch. Then, you cross your legs, lifting your right foot up on your left thigh and your left foot on your right thigh. Yes, this does ensure you maintain a proper spinal position.

If you're not quite that adventurous or flexible, there's an option for you. It comes close to this pose, but isn't exact. The benefits are the same, though. It's called the half lotus. In this posture, you only need to put on foot or the other on top of the opposite thigh.

If neither of these poses appeals to you, you can always sit cross-legged. This is the easiest of the three poses and just may be the one you'd like to start off with. By starting with this simple position, you can actually concentrate on your meditation instead of worrying about whether you're sitting properly.

If even the floor doesn't appeal to you, then just pull up a chair and make yourself at home. But, to effectively meditate, there are a few caveats of how to sit. Ideally, your feet should be on the floor. You should also take note of how our thighs are positioned. They should be parallel to the floor. For some individuals, those who are a bit shorter than the average person or those a bit taller, the proper seating position may present a slight problem. Think about how your thighs are positioned before you settle into a session. If you don't think the position is quite right, you should consider either adopting one of the poses we talked about earlier or trying the lying-down pose.

The lying-down pose is pretty much self-explanatory. You'll meditate on a yoga or pilates mat (or a blanket) on the floor. If this posture is uncomfortable, consider placing a firm cushion under your head. Some persons like to place a book covered with a blanket under their heads. The head then gets the support it may need, and the support is not so hard as to deter you from meditating.

Words to Meditate By: Mantra

This next meditation element isn't actually a required part of every meditation, but it helps to keep your mind focused. It certainly helps when you begin your healing meditation.

This element is a mantra. We've all used the word in our conversations and we have a good idea of what a mantra is, at least in generalized terms. Interestingly, *mantra*, in the ancient Indian language Sanskrit, means "that which frees the mind." In its simplest form, it's a word or even a phrase you chant or recite while you're meditating. A mantra helps you to focus your mind on meditation, keeping some of those stray thoughts at bay.

Some experts recommend you choose a phrase or word with meaning to you. Some people select the word love or joy; others choose a word with an overtly religious meaning. If you're practicing a healing meditation, though, some experts, especially Gabriel Weiss, author of **The Healing Power of Meditation**, suggests a slightly different approach to the selection of a mantra.

Weiss suggests that you adopt a mantra based not on the meaning of the word, but on the *quality of the sound the word makes* when you pronounce it. Probably the most common sound, which has become stereotypically linked with meditation, is the sound, "Ohm." This sound has been the staple mantra for those who meditate for literally thousands of years.

As you begin your healing meditation practice, this may be the mantra you want to adopt. It doesn't necessarily mean you have to stay with it, but it's definitely a great point at which to start. Why not start right now by saying "Ohm" out loud if you're alone. If you have the time, perform this quick and easy illustrative exercise of the power of the "Ohm."

First, sit up straight, preferably in a chair. You're about to begin to chant "Ohm" repeatedly for several minutes, using a deeper than normal voice. It really doesn't matter how loud you repeat this; we're not looking for volume here. You'll see in a few minutes why this isn't a concern.

Next, close your eyes. Inhale slowly and deeply. As you exhale, release this mantra audibly. Hold the "ohm" for as long as you can comfortably do so. The sound should emanate easily and freely from your throat. As you do this, you'll no doubt feel a sense of relaxation--a sensation of freeing of tension. Now you're going to do the same thing, but you're going to chant this sound so low that it can barely be heard, just felt.

These elements of the healing meditation may appear to be disparate right now, but when you blend them into your meditation routine, they create a powerful, synergistic effect.

Chapter 8: Guided Imagery: One Small Habit with Huge, Healthy Consequences

Guided meditation. Guided imagery. Guided visualization.

Whatever you call it, this category of contemplation is the bedrock of any healing meditation program. As you progress on your meditation journey, you'll discover the overriding influence that this seemingly small habit can have on your overall health and well-being.

Guided imagery is different from some other forms of meditation. Most meditation techniques require you to sit still, quiet your mind, and essentially gently sweep all stray thoughts out of the way. With this form, you are, in essence, building a healthier you through visualization.

Seeking Health on All Levels?

The wholeness of health you're seeking may be mental, emotional, spiritual, or physical. Certainly everything you've learned up to this point about healing meditation confirms its powers of supporting good health and providing an improved quality of life. The practice of meditation requires your active involvement. It requires you to not only sit quietly, but also to envision certain scenarios ranging from a relaxing setting in which you may de-stress, to visualizing the destruction of malignant tumors or the creation of healthy cells.

Essentially, it's a system of thoughts created through the suggestions and guidance of an instructor or a recorded script. Through this process, your own imaginary powers propel you into a relaxed, focused state. If you had any doubt up to this point of the intimate link between your mind and your body, you can dispel it now. Guided imagery can provide you with the greatest examples of the exquisite interweaving of the two.

Read the instructions for the following exercise, then try it yourself.

Imagine an orange sitting on a plate in front of you. Imagine the smell of this fruit. See the brilliant color of it. Now, imagine you're picking it up and feeling the texture of the rind. What does it feel like? Peel the orange and, while you're doing this, imagine what it smells like as you break the peel, what the peel feels like, and how much effort is required to pull the rind from the fruit itself. Next, in your mind's eye, split the fruit using the natural wedges on the orange. Now, take a wedge and bite into it. Feel the juice in your mouth. Notice the texture of it.

The Power of the Mind-Body Connection

This experience in guided visualization has caused more than one person to salivate. That's the power of the mind-body connection. It's the same power that can help support healthy blood pressure levels as well as manage other aspects of cardiovascular disease. It's the same awesome power that can help boost your immune system to reduce your chances of catching the flu. It's the same power that can help your body battle cancer cells. The fact of the matter is, healing meditation, especially when expressed through guided imagery, can help you restore and maintain nearly every aspect of your health.

There's plenty of research to back this statement up--too much, in fact, to note here. Below are a few exciting examples. In one study, conducted at Oregon Health and Science University, researchers asked 15 women with either stage I or II breast cancer to participate in hypnotic-guided imagery sessions.

As part of the meditation experience, the women were told to actually see specific protective cells of their immune system, called "natural killer cells," eliminating the destructive cancer cells. All the women were provided with identical recordings of the session. They were to meditate at home three times a week. The study lasted for eight weeks.

The administrators of the study measured the women's immune functions three times throughout the project: at the start, immediately at the end of the eight-week trial, and then three months after that. The researcher then combined the statistics, discovering that the women's natural killer cells had actually increased. Not only that, but a majority of the participants said they experienced less depression.

In another study, conducted in Great Britain, 96 women who had only recently been diagnosed with locally advanced breast cancer were divided into two groups. Both groups were the recipients of conventional cancer therapy and care. But, in addition, one group was asked to practice guided imagery and relaxation training. As you might expect by now, the women in the group who practiced meditation and relaxation techniques were more positive about their quality of life than those who didn't meditate.

The Healing Therapy that Keeps on Healing

It's true: Once the scientific community discovered the power of this incredibly safe complementary treatment, they were astounded at another aspect of its power. The effects of guided imagery stay with you weeks, sometimes months, after you've stopped practicing it.

The results of a study conducted in Korea bear this out. In this project, 60 women, all with breast cancer, were divided into two groups. Researchers instructed one group of 30 women to perform guided visualization. The members of this group were also provided with progressive muscle relaxation training. They were also given the conventional chemotherapy. A second group of 30 females were provided only the traditional chemotherapy for the cancer. The duration of the study was six months.

At the end of the study, those individuals in the group practicing the two complementary therapies experienced less adverse side effects during the chemotherapy treatments. They reported less nausea and vomiting. Not only that, but they reported having less anxiety over the treatments than the other group and were less depressed and irritable.

The Lasting Impact: The Six-Month Follow-Up

While by now those results may not surprise you or the researchers, what the scientists found six months after the project was perhaps the most impressive of all the results. By all accounts, the members of the group who received the complementary treatments of guided visualization and muscle relaxation were still reporting a better quality of life than those who did not meditate.

There are several ways in which you can experience the full potential of this practice. The easiest and quickest way to do this is to go online and discover some of the extremely well-thought out scripts. There are many guided suggestions available which are free and can, at least, give you a taste of what this form of meditation is all about.

Many experts in the field say that your meditation session will be even more rewarding when you're the voice guiding you through the imagery. They recommend you record a script, and then play it back during your meditation. A third method, which is popular as well, is to attend a group meditation session. There, an instructor or therapist leads you and your classmates through a series of visualizations.

Group Guided Meditation: What to Expect

Many individuals hesitate to take this third route even though it's extremely helpful, because of the fear of the unknown. They aren't sure what exactly will happen in a session, so they stay away. Because of this, the following are a few things you can expect to occur if you decide to go to a class.

First, the typical class lasts between 20 and 30 minutes. For the most part, the instructor guides you into a situation or even a location in your mind in which you feel a peaceful and relaxed. Above all, you'll feel secure during this entire process. In addition to the script, there may be gentle, soothing music softly playing in the background, making a truly relaxing atmosphere.

You'll be spending a majority of your time in this session imagining some action. It may be, depending on your purpose and needs, that you'll be asked to see a warm, healing light hovering over the cancer cells in your body. It may also be that you'll be asked to create an object which will "eat away" and eliminate the cells, not unlike the classic video game, Pac-Man.

Or, if you're attending a healing meditation focused on heart disease, you may be asked in some way to visualize the blockages of your arteries disappearing and your arteries themselves widening, allowing more blood to pump through them.

Your instructor may, after the session, ask participants to describe their feelings during the session. You may be asked to detail the types of sensations you experienced. It's not unusual for individuals who are asked to imagine a warm light on the area of their body needing healing to actually feel that warmth. Some individuals will describe how they felt lighter than normal or express their encounter with contentment. Others even say they can feel their bodies growing physically stronger during these sessions.

Surf the Web for Guided Imagery Scripts

If you decide that—at least initially—you'd like to start guided visualization in the privacy of your home, there are many quality resources from which to choose online. One site, which has a large variety of recorded sessions you can access for free, can be found at http://www.fragrantheart.com/cms/free-audio-meditations. Here you'll find guided visualizations not only for cancer and heart disease, but also for stress reduction and pain, to name only a few.

You can find sites like this one simply by typing the words "healing meditation" into your browser. That's how I began when I first made the decision to start my guided imagery program. You may want to narrow your search by typing the disorder you're seeking to heal along with the "healing meditation" or "guided imagery" query.

One of the options we talked about earlier was to record your own voice reading a script for you to listen to later. The following guided meditation can be used for that purpose. You can read it into a recording device yourself, and then play it back when you're ready to meditate. You can also ask someone to read it to you. It's not unusual, additionally, to find a script that's most helpful to you and read that on a regular basis. If you discover one, you may actually have the outline to a script memorized and may not need it to be recited to you. You'll just silently go through the motions.

The following is a generalized guided meditation sample designed for taking you to a more relaxed location in your mind. Your body will naturally follow.

Settle into your meditation position. Get yourself comfortable. Take several deep breaths even before the imagery is introduced. Now, imagine yourself alone on a long stretch of beach. You look up and down the coast. No one else is in sight. You walk down the beach and, as you do, you can feel the warmth of the sun caressing your face. Listen to the gentle lapping of the waves on the shore, the seagulls gliding overhead.

You stop and lie down, taking in the pleasure and relaxing feeling of the warm sand. You close your eyes and remain still for several minutes, breathing in the healing sea air. When you rise, you notice that not far from you is a grove of inviting palm trees. You walk over to them, paying close attention to the leaves rustling in the breeze. As you stand underneath them, you realize the refreshing shade the trees offer.

You continue walking and soon discover a thicket of tropical plants and a path. You're shielded from the sun while in this area, but as you walk through you eventually come to the end. Once you walk into the sun again, you see a tall waterfall. The water is cascading from a cliff into a clear, blue pond.

The waterfall and pond are surrounded by a dazzlingly array of beautifully colored flowers. You can smell the fragrances of the flowers. They're all dancing in the breeze. Then you see them. Butterflies. All sizes. All shapes. They flutter from one flower to the next, lightly dancing around the gorgeous colors.

As you spend more time basking in the sun and the beautiful terrain, you notice your body is getting energized. You're breathing in a sense of renewed energy. You've gained a sense of peace, of serenity. You feel a strength bubbling within you that you haven't felt in a long time. You relish this feeling, enjoying the moment.

As you regain your vitality, you decide without regret to return home, because you know you're returning stronger and healthier. You're also returning more relaxed and peaceful. You also know that you can visit this place anytime you wish. You begin walking away from it all and gently bring yourself out of the meditation.

You Don't Have to Stay Strictly to the Script

As you develop your own guided imagery style, whether its goal is to eliminate cancer cells from your body, ease your joint pain, or lower your blood pressure, you may decide you have a favorite guided script. Use this, by all means, but don't be afraid as you feel to change some aspects around.

As in the meditation provided, you may want to linger longer under the palm trees, or bypass that section altogether, seeing yourself at the waterfall. There is no right or wrong way to create your personalized meditation. If it fits your needs at the time, then it's the perfect practice for you.

When you use guided imagery, you'll receive the best aspects of the ancient healing knowledge as confirmed with the latest scientific research. It doesn't get any better than that.

Chapter 9: The Simple – and Effective – Healing Breath Meditation

Guided imagery is a powerful meditative approach to healing. However, it is not the only approach. The truth is, any form of meditation you select has the potential to restore your health and happiness. The key that unlocks this amazing effect is selecting the technique best suited to your health needs and your lifestyle.

Perhaps you feel as if you can't conjure up the images and scenes requested in a guided visualization session. You may feel you aren't gifted with that innate sense of imagination you may believe it requires. That doesn't mean you have to forego the healing power of this therapeutic activity. There also may be times when you'd prefer to perform a meditation other than the guided variety. By all means, do so, knowing that you're still receiving all the healing benefits of this activity.

You may be surprised at the many versions of meditation that actually exist. The truth is that just about any activity can be transformed into a meditative session when you change your perception about it.

In this chapter, you will be introduced to a simple – yet amazingly effective – technique called breath meditation. This is a meditation you can always return to regardless of the state of your health. You can add to this basic set of instructions later by adding techniques to help you visualize numbers or better focus on your breath. For now, it's a great technique for getting you quickly to the road of healing.

Introduction: The Basic Breathing Meditation

There are a variety of breathing meditations. The difference among them is sometimes as slight as the technique they use to maintain your focus on your breath. Below are the guidelines for a basic breath meditation—nothing fancy, and no clever ways to keep your concentration on your breath. It does, however, represent a fundamental approach to meditation.

Don't let the word "basic" mislead you, though. While the practice may be reduced to its simplest form, its beneficial effects are anything but basic. If this is the only form of meditation you choose to practice in order to receive physical, mental, or emotional healing, it will perform wonders. You'll certainly be amazed at how this small addition to your daily habits can make big inroads into better health.

1. Sit in a chair.

Before you decide on what type of chair in which to sit, consider these few facts. (Didn't know it would get this complicated so soon, did you?) First, you want to ensure your feet will touch the ground (for those height-challenged individuals or children, this may very well be an issue). You'll also want to make sure your thighs are parallel to the floor. This second recommendation affects those who are below average height as well as those who are taller than most of us. In order to obtain the best results, you don't want your thighs slanting down or up.

In order to satisfy these two criteria, you may want to pretend you're Goldilocks – continue to sample chairs until you find the one that's "just right." If you're having an issue finding a chair fitting you properly, you may want to try sitting on the floor (preferably on a yoga mat). When you choose this option, though, use some variation of the cross-legged position we discussed earlier. Just be sure your spine stays straight for the entire session.

If you don't feel comfortable with either of these alternatives, then you might want to consider lying down on your back. It's best if you do this on the floor for the spinal support it provides. You can either place a yoga mat underneath you or a blanket. For head support and comfort, you may want to place a firm pillow under your head as well.

2. Close your eyes.

It's best to get into the habit of closing your eyes when you meditate. This keeps distractions to a minimum. As you become more familiar and accomplished with meditation, you may decide to perform this practice with your eyes open.

When you keep your eyes open, you'll want to focus on one object, usually three or four feet from you. Many individuals choose the flame of a candle. Some choose a random picture on the wall. All this does is to act as an anchor for your focus. You'll eventually decide that meditating with your eyes closed is the best option for you, or you'll discover a style that suits your needs perfectly.

3. Place your hands, palms up, on your lap.

No doubt you've seen the classic meditative pose in which the thumb and the second finger of the meditator are touching. When you place your hands in any specific position as you perform this activity, it's referred to as a mudra.

While this can certainly work as an effective aid for some people in keeping their mind focused, it's not necessary to do this. You can receive all the wonderful rewards of meditation, simply by placing your hands on your thighs.

4. Take a few minutes to relax your muscles.

Yes, I do know that's one of the goals of meditation and it will eventually occur as you meditate. It's also good, however, to attempt to relax as much as possible prior to your actual session. In essence, you're making yourself especially receptive to the eventual peaceful consequences of meditation. Many individuals call this short and simple routine centering.

5. Place your attention on your abdomen.

This is the hallmark characteristic of a breathing meditation: attention to the abdominal portion of your body. Specifically, you'll want to focus your energy on the portion of your stomach that's about two inches above your navel. It lies along the vertical midsection of your body.

There's no need to physically look down to view this. Simply use your mind's eyes in placing your focus here.

6. Observe the physical movement of your breath.

You'll observe this more or less naturally as your attention turns to your abdomen. You'll want to take note of your stomach's rhythmic rising and falling. There are several aspects you need to pay close attention to. First, remember to breathe from your diaphragm. As you inhale as well as exhale, you'll want to keep these breaths extended for as long as possible.

Do this for 10 consecutive breaths, maintaining your focus on your breath for the entire time. Counting your breath is a great way to do this. Count each complete exhale and inhale as one full breath. Start at 1, making your way to 10. If at any time during this process thoughts intrude and you lose your place, start over at one. Don't worry if you have to start over several times in order to complete 10 consecutive breaths. Especially as you begin, you'll find this seemingly simple exercise to be challenging.

7. Take 10 – again.

Once you've successfully completed 10 consecutive breaths without stray thoughts intruding and distracting you, repeat it. Take another 10 consecutive breaths. For the second set, though, you'll silently repeat a one-word mantra of your choice. This may be "ohm," the traditional sound associated with meditation. It may also be any word of your choosing, especially one that carries a meaning for you. You may choose "love," "peace," or any other word.

8. Observe your meditation session as if you were a detached, impassive observer.

No, this isn't one of the easiest aspects of this practice. It is, though, one which will eventually bring you many benefits. It's also one of the most difficult aspects to try to explain to someone. You'll want to view the rising and falling of your abdomen as if it were occurring to someone else.

This means you don't judge anything about it. You don't try to figure out if this is what the movement is really *supposed to be*, or if it's healthy, or if it's somehow even making a difference in your life. Observe. Only observe.

9. Observe your thoughts from a detached viewpoint.

Use the same process you did with your abdomen and your breath with your thoughts. Observe them impassively as if they belonged to someone else. Of course, your goal is to free your mind from thinking, but that's like asking a bird not to fly.

The best any of us can hope for most of the time is to gently sweep them away. In the meantime, view any lingering thoughts as if you were viewing another person's passing ruminations. Don't spend time trying to decide why they appeared or chastise yourself for thinking them. Don't give them any more energy than they deserve right now – which is none.

Eventually, your mind will realize that it's not making any headway trying to obstruct your quiet time with intrusive thoughts. As you gain experience, the number of thoughts floating through your mind will lessen. But keep in mind, they'll never disappear totally.

10. Remember, you're living in the present.

One of the remarkable abilities of meditation is the potential it has to keep you firmly locked in the present. This happens automatically as you focus on your breath and allow your thoughts (which usually concern the past or the future) to float by without you encouraging their presence.

11. Label the moment.

It's not unusual to talk about labeling something as some aspect of judging it. We label things everyday as good or bad, right or wrong, happy or sad. This isn't at all what is meant when you label a moment, meditatively speaking. It means you're recognizing it and simply *identifying it*. To label something, you simply make a mental note of it. For example, you'll make a note mentally each time your breath falls and each time it rises. That's what is meant by labeling.

This simple meditation holds the key to your healing as surely as any of the others presented here. If you occasionally find you can't fit your regular guided imagery meditation or your normal walking meditation into your day, you can at least find five minutes to close your eyes and become aware of your breath and the present.

Chapter 10: Exercise Your Mind And Body: The Walking Meditation

There are several variations of walking meditations. You may be familiar with the type in which you move slowly (sometimes excruciatingly slowly), observing every step and labeling it. In the one presented here, you can walk for fitness as well as relaxing purposes, combining the best of both worlds: meditation and physical exercise.

Like the slow movement walk, this practice requires you to focus all of your attention on your body's movements – at least a certain aspect of them. The first rule of thumb is to avoid talking and thinking during this time. Dedicate this time to walking only. If you choose to walk with another person, it would be perfect if both of you were doing so as a meditation.

Your goal is to maintain the focus on your body for the length of your walk. Depending on your level of fitness and your powers of focus, start by walking 15 minutes daily at least three times a week. If you find that this is too long – either because of physical reasons or your attention span – then reduce the amount of time. You may want to try 10 minutes to start – or even less.

The key is to perform the walking meditation as best as you can. You don't have to achieve a preconceived external standard. As you improve both your health and your focus, you can always increase the length of the sessions. The following are several general guidelines to keep uppermost in your mind as you walk.

1. Keep your spine straight as you prepare your body for the meditation.

Just as in the breathing meditation, where you kept your spine straightened to facilitate the natural flow of your breath and energy to all areas of your body, you'll want to do the same here. As you prepare to walk, you'll want to try to keep your head parallel with the ground. If you find yourself looking down, raise your head and look straight ahead of you. Do the same if you realize you're looking up consistently as well. You'll also want to keep your shoulders back. In essence, you want to walk just the way your parents always urged you to do – with proper posture.

2. Focus on one area of your body.

As we progress in the guidelines, we'll talk about other objects you can focus on while you walk. But as you begin your routine and it's still new to you, try to keep your concentration on one portion of your body. Perhaps the most logical choice, as well as the most common, is focusing on the movement of your feet.

If you select this, you'll make yourself aware of the bottom of your feet as they touch and gently grip the ground with each step. In fact, that's the key: to become exceedingly attuned to each step you take.

If you prefer not to focus your awareness on your feet, consider concentrating instead on the sensations created in your legs when you walk. Another option would be to place your attention on your fingers. Notice how they feel as they swing through the air, with the breeze hitting them.

There are any number of aspects of your walk that you can deliberately turn your attention to. If you decide on another area of your body instead of the ones mentioned here, by all means do so.

3. Relish every step you take.

Sure, I've already suggested that you pay attention to each and every step. But more than that, take *enjoyment* in those steps. Walking is something that most of us take for granted. This meditation is the time to realize what your body is feeling and actually enjoy the activity. Your meditation won't be successful if you're complaining about the physical activity itself while you're walking. It's this mindful enjoyment that can help banish your sadness, anger, despair, depression, and even help alleviate your physical ailments.

4. Pay attention to your breath.

There's no way to get around it. If you're meditating, you're naturally attuned to your breathing. Breath is, after all, the key to all effective meditation sessions – even your walking regimen. Adopt a detached observational outlook on it. Focus on it, but in no way try to control it.

You may want to time your steps so they are in some way aligned with your breathing pattern. You can also count the number of steps you take as you inhale and exhale. This helps to keep you focused on the movements of your body, concentrated on your breath, and squarely centered in the present moment.

5. Design your own walking routine.

The key to transforming an activity into a habit is by doing something you love. Don't force a routine into your walking meditation that you're not comfortable with. In fact, don't even continue this particular practice if don't think you can ever learn to enjoy walking. Don't brood over the fact that you believe you should be doing this. Meditation is designed to relieve stress, not to create more of it in your life.

If counting breaths, for example, or focusing your body becomes monotonous, then develop a ritual that will keep your interest. You may want to recite a favorite poem or even adopt a mantra you can say while you walk. Instead of focusing on their bodies, some individuals prefer to turn that detached observational viewpoint outward and study the trees or flowers. The beauty of this activity is that you can do it practically anywhere. You can enter a park and begin your meditation or you can walk down a quiet country lane or even in a lush wooded area.

The only place you probably wouldn't try to meditate is along busy city streets. Don't attempt – especially as you start off – to walk on the sidewalks of New York City, for example. You're not going to discover much peace and you certainly won't develop any sense of serenity doing this.

An increasingly popular walking location is in a labyrinth. This is a circular path specifically designed for meditation. These have been used for thousands of years. You enter at a point and follow the path as it circles around several times to eventually lead you to the center of the circle. Then you walk out along the same path that led you in. It's not at all a maze where you have to guess which routes to take.

The labyrinth has been used as an effective tool to enhance meditation for hundreds of years.

You may find it suits your needs. If you're interested in finding one near you, visit http://labyrinthlocator.com/.

A Rainy Day Option

Walking meditations are best enjoyed outside. As you commune with nature, you may begin to truly feel united with your surroundings. You can be quite sure though that there will be some days where you won't be able to enjoy this activity outside due to less than desirable weather conditions.

This doesn't mean you have to forego your meditation for that day. You'll just need to make adjustments. Consider walking inside. Undoubtedly you'll need to slow your pace some and do some planning ahead of time. One of the ways you can still walk and meditate is by choosing a large room. This may be in your home or perhaps in your office or other area. Many schools open portions of their buildings to walkers at various times of the day. You may have one in your area.

After you choose your room, you'll begin to walk as close to the perimeter of it as you can. Start out as close to the walls as possible. Each time you inhale, take a step. Each time you exhale, take another step. As you complete your first rotation of the room, go around it again.

This time though, move away from the walls a bit. Repeat this circular walking motion through as many increments as possible. Always move away from the wall a little more with each complete rotation.

What you're doing, in effect, is creating your own labyrinth. You can complete the meditation once you're in the center of the room, or you can walk in the opposite circular direction from the center to the walls.

A walking meditation can be a powerful and unique source of healing. Don't overestimate the fact that just being outdoors and experiencing the air and taking in the beauty of nature can help heal you. If you're physically capable of walking, even short distances, you should seriously consider performing this – even if it isn't your main form of meditation.

Chapter 11: One Effective Approach to Pain Management: Meditation

Pain… probably the most common ailment in society today. Ironically, it is probably the most difficult ailment for professional health-care providers to treat. The presence of pain in the human body is a complex affair.

No two individuals feel pain in quite the same way. What one person describes as merely an annoyance, another may label as intensely agonizing. Who is right? They both are. That's one of the dilemmas with pain management. Another problem lies in the quantity and quality of training that the majority of doctors receive in this area. Many are not equipped to address pain – especially chronic pain – except through the use of prescription drugs.

This isn't just one person's opinion or the results of casual observations. A growing chorus of doctors is calling for an investigation into more effective ways to treat chronic pain. Currently, there are more than 70 million Americans who suffer from this problem. The treatment of pain, along with time lost from work for many individuals, costs the economy about $100 billion annually, according to an article in *The New York Times* several years ago.

The situation is complicated even further because of the government's strict standards when it comes to prescribing pain-killing, narcotic drugs. Doctors who appear to be handing out too many prescriptions can be the target of investigations.

What This Means to You

If you suffer from chronic pain, you already know that this can translate into visiting doctor after doctor, many of whom suggest surgery or other forms of treatments. Many of these treatments can be ineffective as well as expensive. If you've visited enough doctors, some may even try to talk you out of your pain, telling you that it's all in your head.

There's still one more piece of the pain puzzle that appears to elude many of us. While we endure this pain and try palliative remedies to rid our bodies of it (or at the very least, reduce it), many of us still have a nagging question. What does the pain mean? What is your body trying to tell you? Many individuals fear that this unexplained and seemingly untreatable pain is the harbinger of some disastrous medical diagnosis.

For all of these reasons, many individuals are turning to meditation to help not only assuage the pain itself, but to allay some the fears that naturally accompany it. Dr. Gabrielle Weiss suggests in his book that the subject separates the physical sensation of pain from the fear of its ultimate meaning. This is only done, he says, by sitting quietly in the present moment – that is through meditation.

Pain Lessened in a Surprisingly Short Amount of Time

Dr. Weiss is talking about a concept greater than what he's experienced in his practice. Several studies confirm that meditation, at the very least, can help lessen your body's perception of pain.

In one study, participants agreed to undergo getting mildly burned in order to test the hypothesis.

The research took place at the Wake Forest University School of Medicine where 15 individuals agreed to be burned mildly not just once, but twice. They were subjected to the identical pain stimulus, a 120-degree burn. The first burn was administered right before they began a series of four 20-minute meditation sessions. The second injury was sustained following the sessions. On both occasions, they were asked to rate their perception of the pain.

The participants rated the second burn--the one following the meditation session--as being overall 57 percent less unpleasant and 40 percent less intense. The researchers noted that this notable drop in pain-relieving performance outstripped other projects seeking to quantify pain relief. Meditation proved more beneficial than placebo pills and hypnosis. Meditation, in this study, also proved to be more effective than prescription pain-killing drugs, including morphine.

The truly astounding outcome of this study, though, was how little meditation was necessary in order to begin feeling its benefits. In effect, it only took 80 minutes of quieting the mind to yield those incredible results.

Of course there's no guarantee that once you meditate you'll be sensing the effects of this therapy that quickly. But if nothing else, this practice can help allay your fears, calm your mind, and perhaps even alleviate a portion of any depression you may be feeling due to the pain.

Below are a set of guidelines you can use to start. As you feel more comfortable in this practice, you'll soon find yourself making personal adjustments in your routine – adjustments, no doubt, that will eventually trigger even better results.

1. Start with a breathing technique.

Get comfortable in a meditative position, whether it's some form of sitting or lying down. To start with, you may not want to consider a walking meditation. You can, however, add this later. Focus on your breath as discussed previously. It's recommended that you perform this as an introduction to your session. Its primary purpose is to help to calm your fears about the pain and its origins.

2. Use the pain as a tool to direct your breathing.

In a nutshell, you should attempt to "breathe with the pain." This may come as a surprise to you and may even seem counterintuitive. It may even be the very last thing you want to do. The idea is not to meditate it away, as you might expect, but to be fully and detachedly aware of the pain. When some instructors direct their students to do this, they tell them to become friends with the pain. While that may be difficult, at least initially, it is very good advice.

The most effective approach to this is to inhale. As you do that, imagine you are actually breathing in through the most painful portion of your body. This takes courage on your part, because in essence you're opening yourself up to becoming vividly aware of the pain.

As you exhale, you'll target the same portion of your body. But now imagine you're breathing out through a hole in that area. As you breathe out, purposely see yourself releasing pain and any related tension through this opening.

You'll eventually be able to feel distinct changes in the intensity and quality of your pain as you "breathe it out of your body." This exhalation portion of the breathing also gives you a sense of peace and calmness.

3. Focus on areas of your body that are not hurting you.

This is called modeling meditation. Its purpose is quite clear. In order to achieve your goal of reducing your pain, you'll focus your attention on a pain-free area. Think about the efficiency at which this body part is working and how it feels not to be in pain.

For example, if you have one knee that is hurting but your other is not, then focus your thoughts on how marvelous the other one is feeling and how effectively it's functioning. What you're doing, in effect, is giving the area of your body that hurts a good role model to follow. Don't laugh until you've tried it.

In more serious terms, you're focusing your attention not on your pain, but rather on your *health*. Very often what we focus on in our lives expands. In effect, you've set your sights on expanding your health through this technique.

This meditative exercise is asking quite a bit from anyone who has lived with near constant pain. It may very well be that you'll need to get accustomed with a basic meditation routine before you step into this one.

Keep in mind that while this particular technique was designed with pain management in mind, any form of meditation will contribute to your healing. Meet your pain where you're most comfortable. You don't need to befriend it immediately. Simply meditating will help you physically, mentally, and emotionally in handling your chronic physical problem and any accompanying unwanted emotional side effects.

Chapter 12: Laughing Your Way to Health: Laughter Meditation

Laughter and meditation combined into one experience? Does that even seem possible? It may seem counterintuitive, given everything you've already learned about effective healing meditation, but the approach exists.

Not only that, but according to some experts, it's one of the most powerful meditation techniques available. Think back to the last time you enjoyed a hearty belly laugh. You may have felt it had a cathartic effect. That's not unusual. Now, consider this scenario. You're at one of the most solemn moments of your life – your wedding vows or worse yet, the funeral of a loved one – when something strikes you as funny. You can't help but laugh.

When laughter does break out in these situations, people inevitably describe it as relieving the tension. Just a phrase, you may say, but it actually comes closer to the truth than you may think. Current research points to these beneficial changes in your physiology when you engage in sustained laughter. It can:

- Reduce your perceived stress level
- Increase the functioning of your immune system
- Lower cholesterol

- Normalize blood pressure level
- Relieve anxiety
- Ease depression
- Boost your brain functioning
- Enhance your decision-making powers
- Increase your overall sense of happiness

Nearly 50 years ago, Norman Cousins pioneered the use of laughter as a healing tool. While he didn't perform a formal laughter meditation, he did experiment by testing his hypothesis that laughter could assuage the joint pain he was feeling.

Afflicted by a disease called ankylosing spondylitis, a widespread inflammation of the joints of the spine as well as those between the spine and pelvis, Cousins, who had no medical training, presented his ideas on the curative natural ability of laughter to his doctor. His doctor agreed to the idea. Cousins wanted to see if laughter – a positive emotional outlet – could ease the pain. From his hospital bed, he watched reruns of the *Candid Camera* television show, as well as the Marx Brothers' movies.

As Cousins detailed in his book, ***Anatomy of an Illness***, the experiment worked. "I made the joyous discovery," he wrote, "that ten minutes of genuine belly laughter had an anesthetic effect and would give me at least two hours of pain-free sleep." When the effects of the laughter wore off, he explained that he would watch another round of comedy.

Laughing Your Way to Health?

Probably up until this point, you never even thought about using the same laughter that dissolves the stress in the room – or eased Cousins's pain – to help provide your body with a form of natural physiological relief.

This type of meditation is, according to meditation experts, one of the simplest techniques to use. But more than that, laughing is one of the few physical actions which involve your body as well as your emotions. Through this much overlooked act, you surrender yourself to the present moment. Really, isn't that what meditation is all about?

Any time of the day is a good time to laugh. If you decide to perform this meditation in the morning, you're preparing yourself for a day highlighted with joy. When you perform it in the evening, you will employ a natural way to relax after a tense day. But more than that, this form of meditation shows you just how absurd life can be at times. It encourages you to laugh in the face of your troubles and to stop taking everything so seriously – including yourself.

You may decide laughing is not a suitable meditation to perform as part of your established, regular meditation routine. However, it may be the perfect addition to bring out when nothing else seems to be working in your life.

So how do you start? Here are three quick steps to guide you through an effective laughing meditation. You decide on the length of time you perform each step. Most experts recommend each portion can be performed for as little as five minutes or as long as 20. As with any meditation, it's probably best you start by trying it for a minimum amount of time, then work your way to longer sessions as you become accustomed to it.

1. Stretch

Yes, that's correct. Your first act is not to sit comfortably in a chair as with all the other forms of meditation. You're going to stretch your entire body. Have you ever seen a cat stretch when he wakes up from a nap? He stretches long and puts quite of bit of effort into it.

Begin by stretching your hands and your feet. Then stretch through the rest of your body. After you've done that, stretch the muscles of your face by yawning and making silly faces.

2. Laugh

Just start with the laughter immediately after you've completed your stretching warm up. Do whatever you can do stimulate your laughter. Visualize a personal humorous situation. Recall one of your favorite jokes or a comedy routine you love.

Once the laughter gets started, allow it to grow. You may feel awkward at first; that's not unusual. You may require some time and practice in adjusting to laughing for no apparent reason – other than your health, of course.

Don't ever try to contain your laughter. Include as many guffaws, chortles, and giggles as you can. It may be that as you start the laughing portion of this meditation, it may only last five minutes. That's fine. As you become accustomed and feel more comfortable with purposely calling forth laughter, you'll naturally be able to sustain it for longer periods of time.

3. Sit still and experience the silence

The final segment is a traditional meditation session. Sit or lie quietly. Still your mind and focus on your breath. Should any stray thoughts float your way, gently sweep them out of your mind. For full details on this portion of the meditation, consult the chapter describing breath meditation.

You may perform this last portion for five to 20 minutes. Don't rush this segment. It's just as important and vital for the healing process.

You may discover laughing meditation to be a most effective – and delightful – approach to healing your body. Who knows? In the process, you may also come to personally confirm what the *Readers' Digest* has been telling us for so long: laughter really is the best medicine.

Conclusion

Meditation of any kind can be a source of healing. If nothing else, the silence of 20 minutes helps to mitigate stress and your reaction to events around you. If meditation does nothing else for you, it'll help you face the world from a more serene outlook.

But more than that, a reduction of stress has been noted in medical study after medical study to be beneficial to your physiology as well. To put it in plain English, meditation can positively affect your physical well-being. From heart disease to cancer to depression, stress has been proven to be an aggravating contributor. Eliminate the stress – even a portion of stress – in the equation, and the odds of your dealing with these diseases increases.

Whether you choose the classic breath meditation, walking meditation, guided imagery or any of the techniques from the book (or a combination of them), you'll discover a whole new world opening up to you. If you're already battling any of these health issues, then you'll discover that the meditation helps to assuage your health issue. Perhaps, though, the most amazing aspect of this complementary approach to healing is that it's without any adverse side effects, unlike many prescription medications.

That's not to say you should toss your prescription drugs into the garbage the moment you meditate. But don't be surprised that, with time, you'll be able to slowly reduce the amount of medications you may be taking. The other serendipitous side effect is to see the look on your health care provider's face when he asks how you managed the improved health. And don't be concerned, if at least initially, he refuses to believe you.

Meditation for healing the body is now more popular than ever before. With the rise of integrative medical services, more physicians are recommending it – and more people are giving it a try. So, what do you have to lose? Give healing meditation an honest try. It just might prove to be one of the best health-related moves you've ever made.

**Visit
EmpowermentNation.com
to view other fantastic books,
sign up for book alerts, giveaways, and
updates!**